The Authentic® Greek Salad Recipe

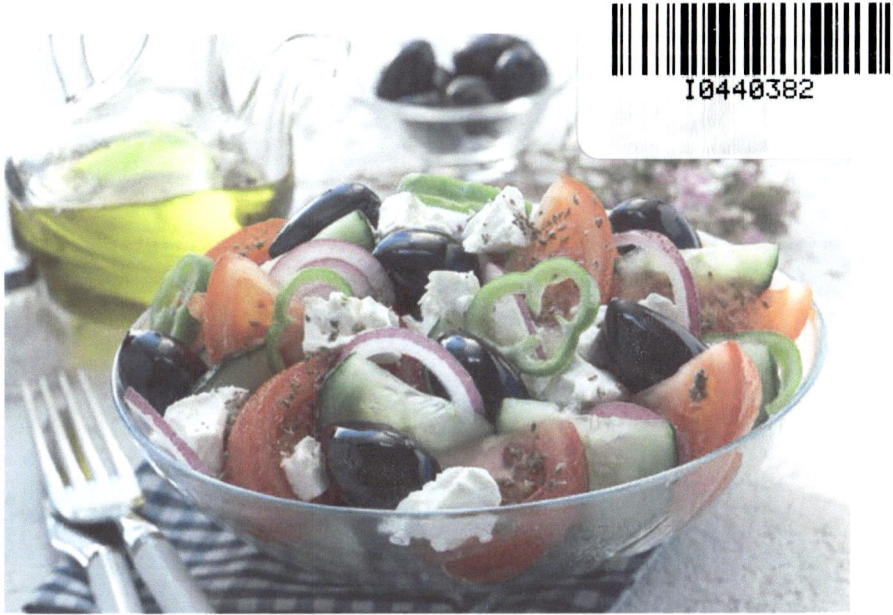

This book is proudly brought to you by:

Lazaros Georgoulas

Researcher and Author

lazageo@gmail.com

Visit my Amazon Author Central:

http://amazon.com/author/lazarosgeorgoulas

ISBN-13: 978-1499325096

ISBN-10: 1499325096

Disclaimer: This recipe of the famous (and nutritious) Greek Salad presented in this book, is the same recipe that verified Greek restaurants are using in their cuisines.

This book may contain promotional materials aiming to further enhance the research possibilities of the reader on subjects related to the Greek Salad recipe, nutrition, diets etc.

Printed by CreateSpace, an Amazon.com company

Table of Contents

ONLINE PROMOTIONS

(SELECTED CAREFULLY – I WILL KEEP THE ORDERS VALID FOR AS LONG AS I CAN!)

Herbs, **oils** and other **aphrodisiacs!** Highly recommended, please visit this address (URL):

http://hyperdeals.biz/go/17/

Learn all the secrets of Wines. Become a wine expert. Go here:

http://hyperdeals.biz/go/14/

Introduction to Greek Salad

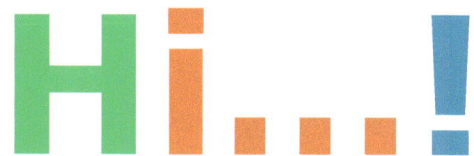

Again, thanks for acquiring this eye-opening mini book...

This shows you are a person who cares about their nutrition.

You must also be among those people who are aware of <u>the importance of food</u> in our life... ;)

Greek cuisine is one of the healthiest because it based on olive oil.

Along with the main dish, Greeks add the famous Greek Salad full of fresh, reviving vegetables, energizing Feta Cheese, herbs and of course the King of Greek Cuisine... Olive oil on top of the rest of the ingredients.

If you visit the various territories in Greece you will find a lot of variations of the authentic Greek Salad recipe.

Others use green cucumbers, others place only tomatoes and fresh or dried onions etc.

In this book you will find the **Authentic Greek Salad Recipe** as presented only by <u>original</u> and **<u>verified</u>** <u>Greek restaurants and taverns</u> in Greece and other places around the world.

A plate of Greek salad can act as a full meal because it contains <u>all you need</u> to be energized and perform your 100%

So, you can add this salad to your nutrition as a single dish or along with a main dish and you will notice the tremendous boost that it will give to your health and to your overall performance in every day life... ;)

Ancient Greeks were not fools.

They knew how to combine what nature and their land had to offer.

And they did it in a magnificent way creating a recipe that stood along the ages. Today it is modernized but the powerful "ancient touch" remains.

Again, the whole secret lies in the use of **olive oil**. I suggest you add it to your cooking habits too.

I don't have to state the benefits of **olive oil** or the rest of the ingredients, you can search online or ask an expert and see what they'll tell you.-

So, without further delay let's see the <u>authentic</u> recipe of the famous Greek salad...

■ ■ ■

The
Authentic
Recipe Of
The Famous
Greek Salad

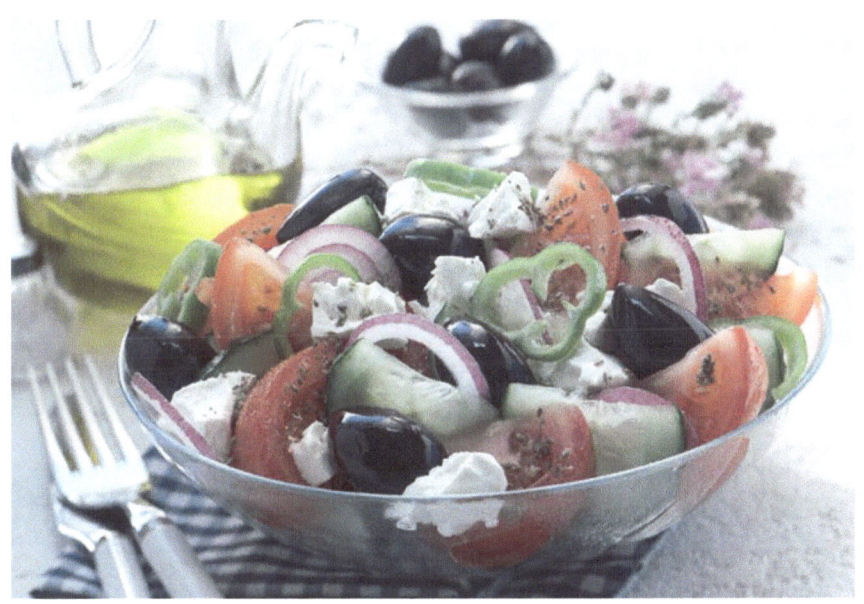

<u>INGREDIENTS</u> (2 people):

- **2 fresh normal sized tomatoes**

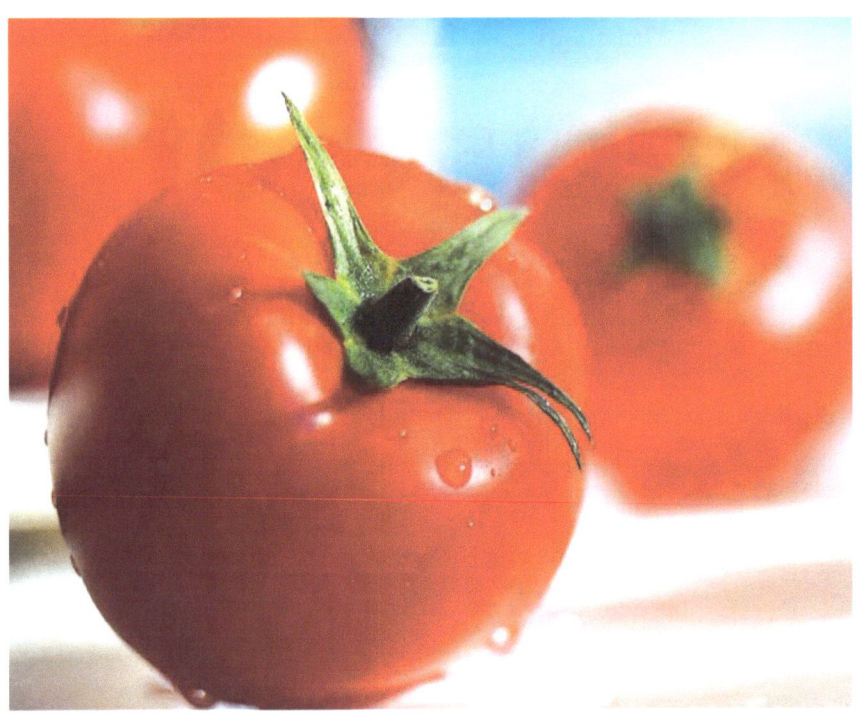

YOUR NOTES...:

_____
_____
_____
_____
_____
_____
_____

- **1 fresh medium sized green cucumber**

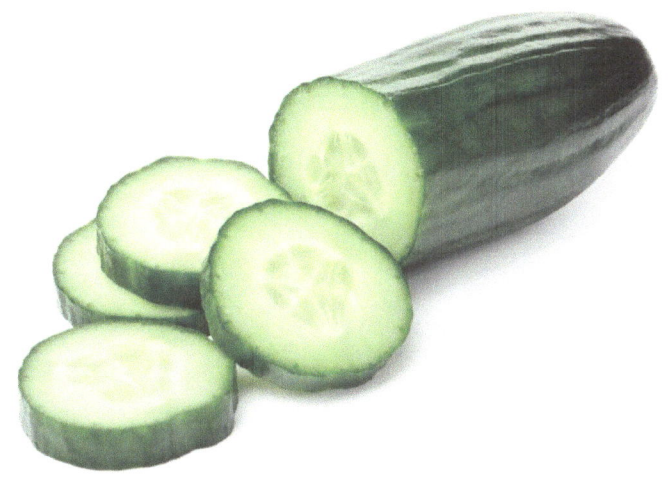

YOUR NOTES...:

_____

_____

_____

_____

_____

_____

_____

_____

_____

_____

- **A few black olives (Experiment and add as many as you like, not too many!)**

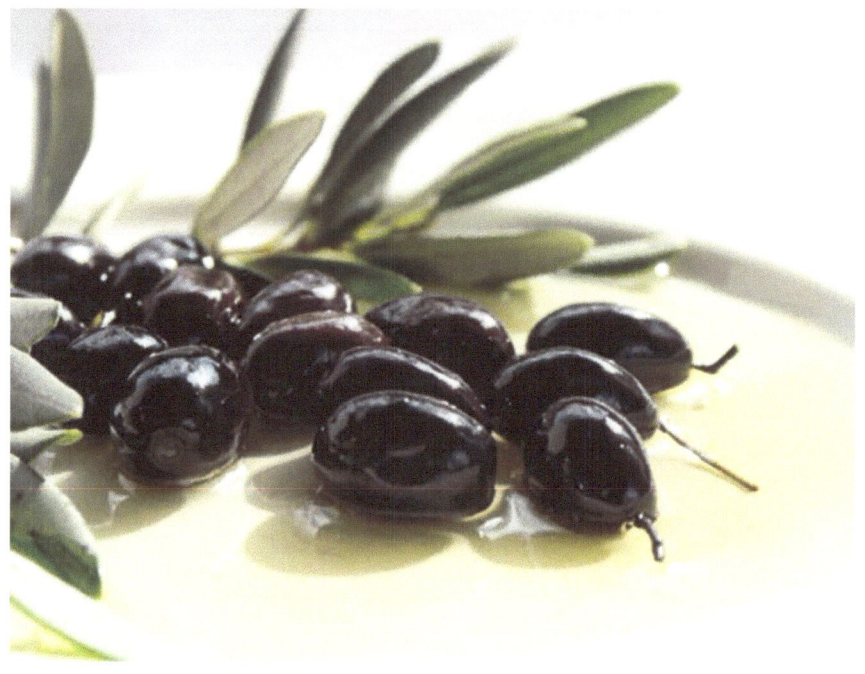

YOUR NOTES...:

_____

_____

_____

_____

_____

_____

_____

_____

- **1 big piece (or 2!) of traditional Feta Cheese (Greeks export tons of it worldwide. If you can't find it, replace it with white goat's cheese or sheep's cheese, not traditional cow's cheese)**

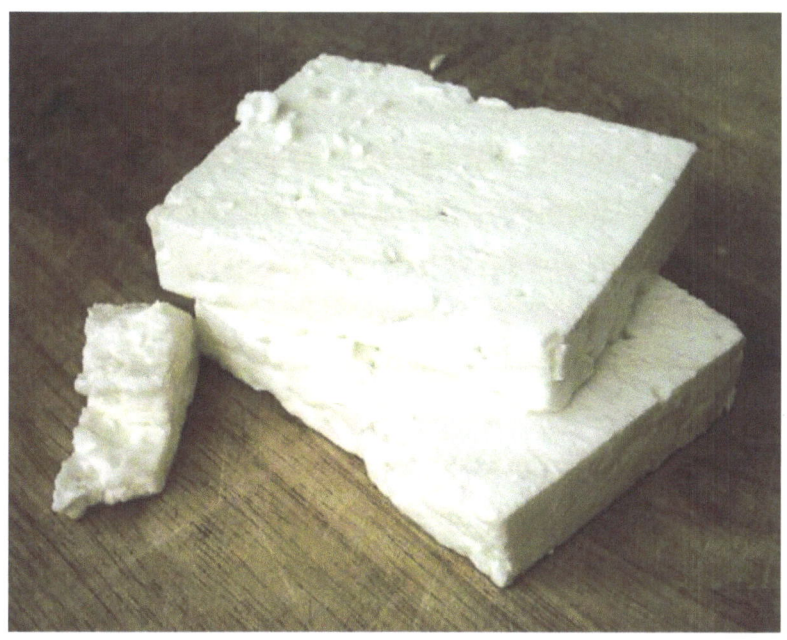

YOUR NOTES...:

_____
_____
_____
_____

- **Fresh (green) or dried onion** or both (add as much as you like. Onion strengthens the heart)

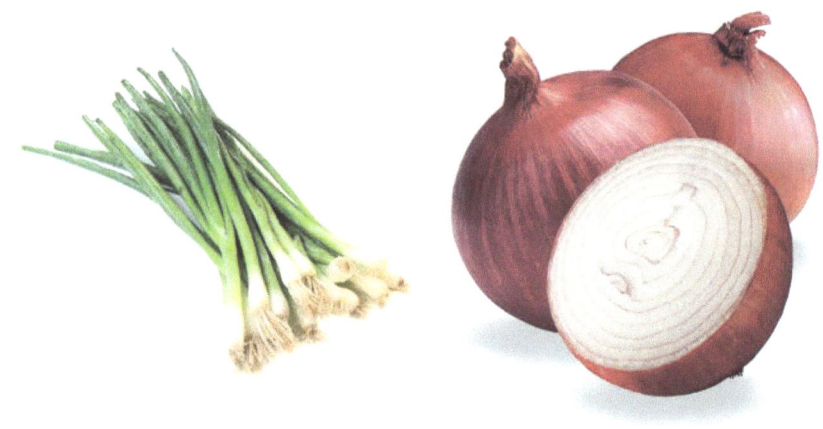

YOUR NOTES...:

_____
_____
_____
_____
_____
_____
_____
_____
_____
_____

- **1 small green pepper**

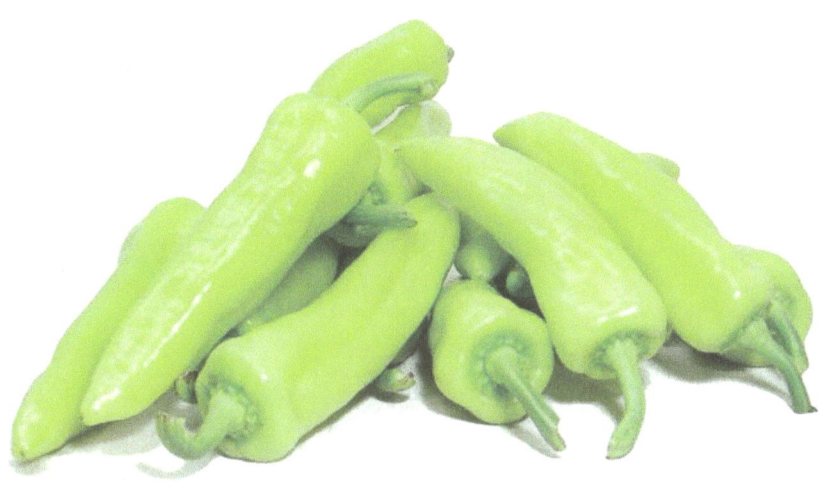

YOUR NOTES...:

_____
_____
_____
_____
_____
_____
_____
_____
_____
_____

- **1 small chilli pepper** (Red. That is, if you like hot stuff in your meals)

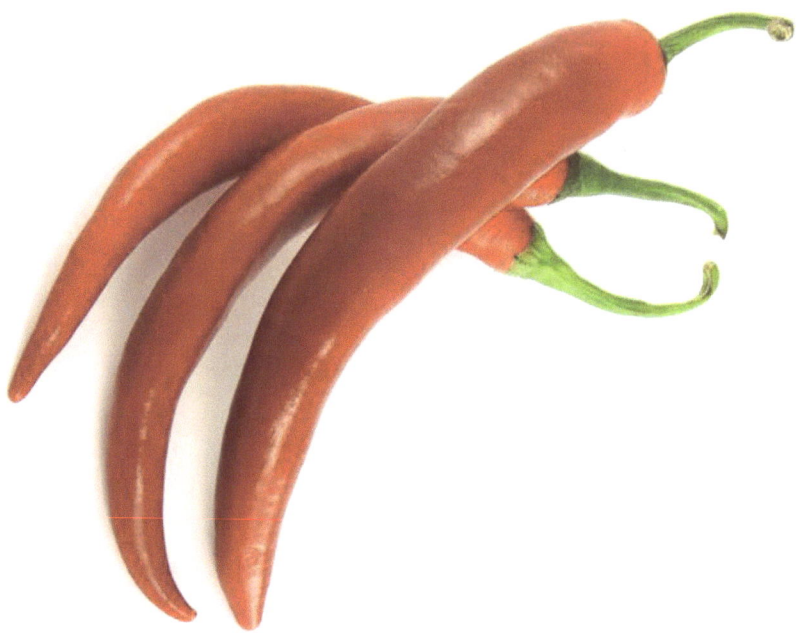

YOUR NOTES...:

_____

_____

_____

_____

_____

_____

_____

_____

- **Salt** (coarse salt recommended. Experiment and add as much as you like)

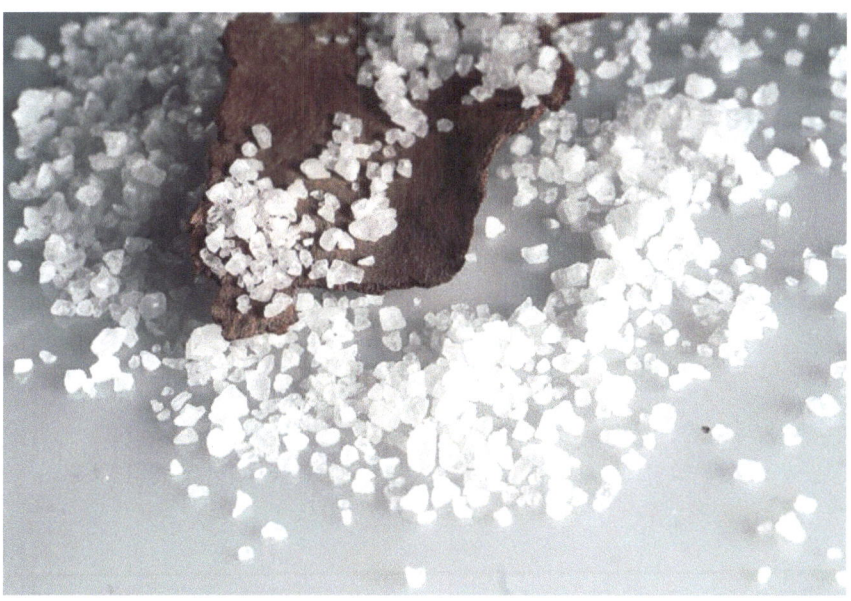

YOUR NOTES...:

_____

_____

_____

_____

_____

_____

_____

_____

- **Some fresh or dried oregano (Experiment and add as much as you like)**

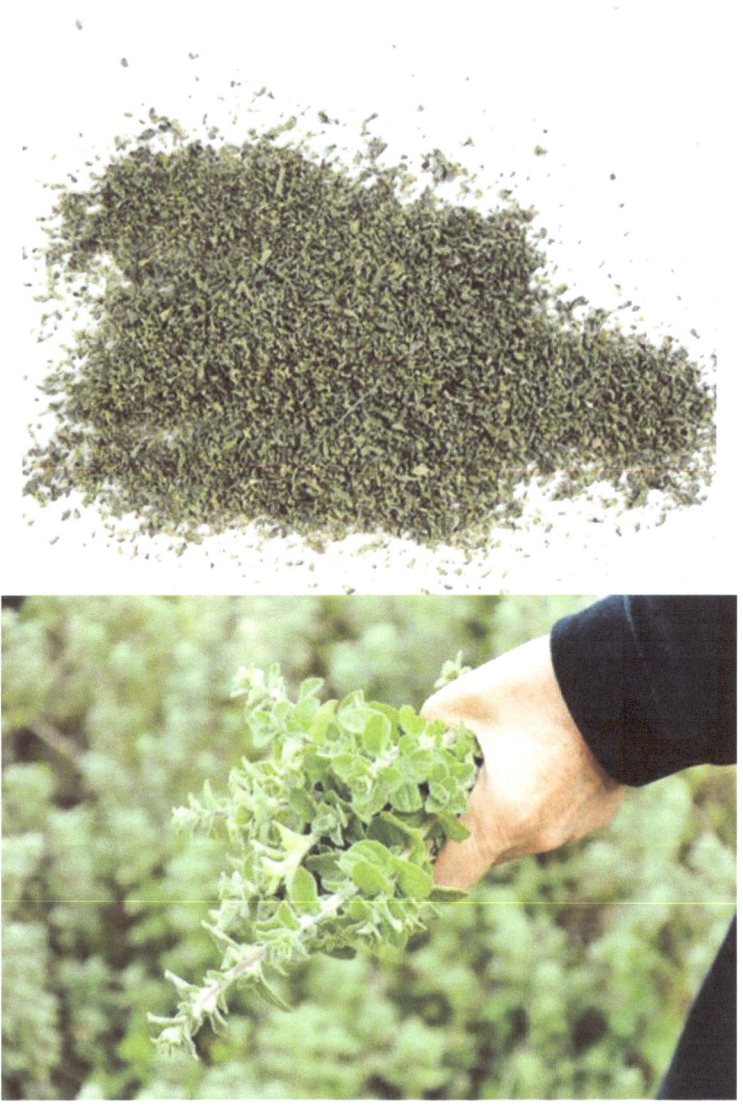

- ## 1 tea spoon of vinegar

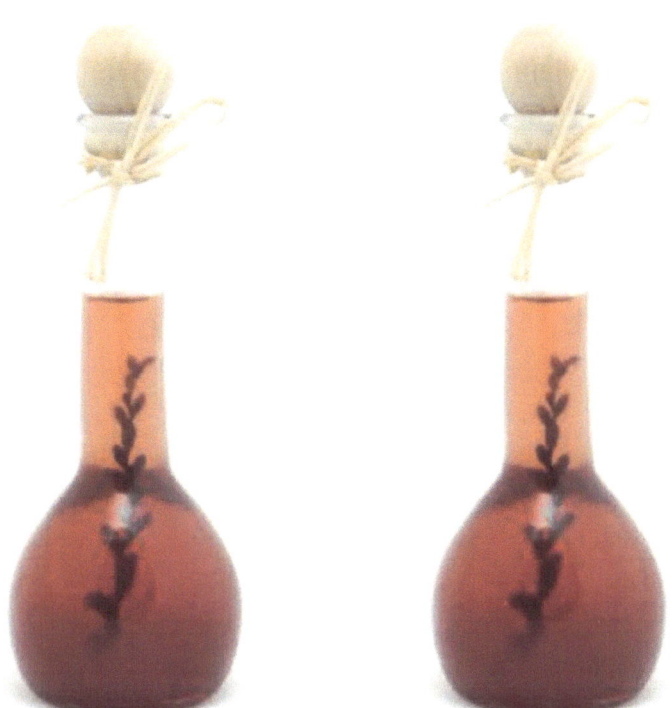

YOUR NOTES...:

_____

_____

_____

_____

_____

_____

_____

_____

- **And finally the King of this dish.** ½ tea cup (or more) of Extra Virgin Olive Oil!

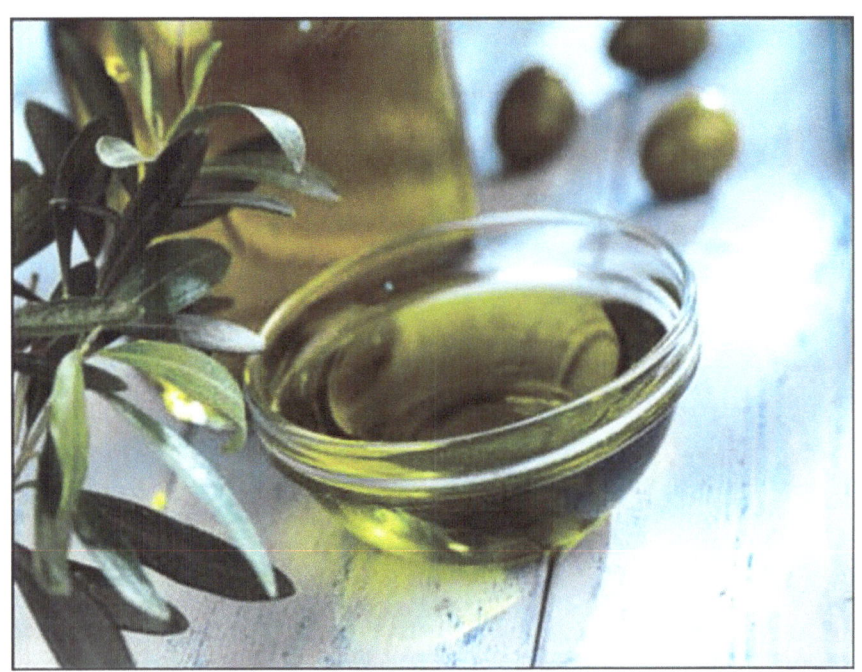

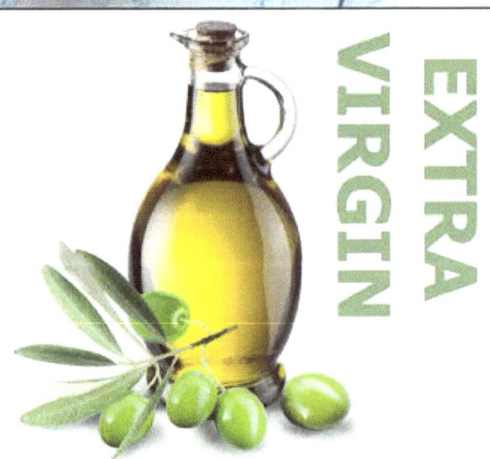

And that's all! You can find most of these in every grocery store or supermarket...

BUT...

Let's see how you can prepare this powerful dish which by the way is an ideal meal for every time of the day.-

YOUR NOTES...:

_____

_____

_____

_____

_____

_____

_____

PREPARATION:

First of all, have all the ingredients ready.

The Preparation of the Greek Salad is sooooo amazingly simple but you have to place the ingredients in the right order (secret)... ;)

First, You cut the vegetables, apart from the olives, into small pieces (you should experiment and decide which piece size you like in your salad for each vegetable)

Then you place them in the salad plate. Tomatoes, Cucumber, Onion(s), Olives, Peppers,.

You add the Vinegar, the Salt and then the Oregano.

Then you take the Feta Cheese and either cut it in small equal pieces, or rub it with your hand and spread it in the salad plate...

Last but not least, you have to add the magic ingredients that boosts the rest.

You guessed well it's the Extra Virgin Olive Oil and you add it as the last ingredient...

Then you mix all the ingredients together until the Vinegar disinfects the vegetables and the olive oil is well spread among all the ingredients.

And there you have it!

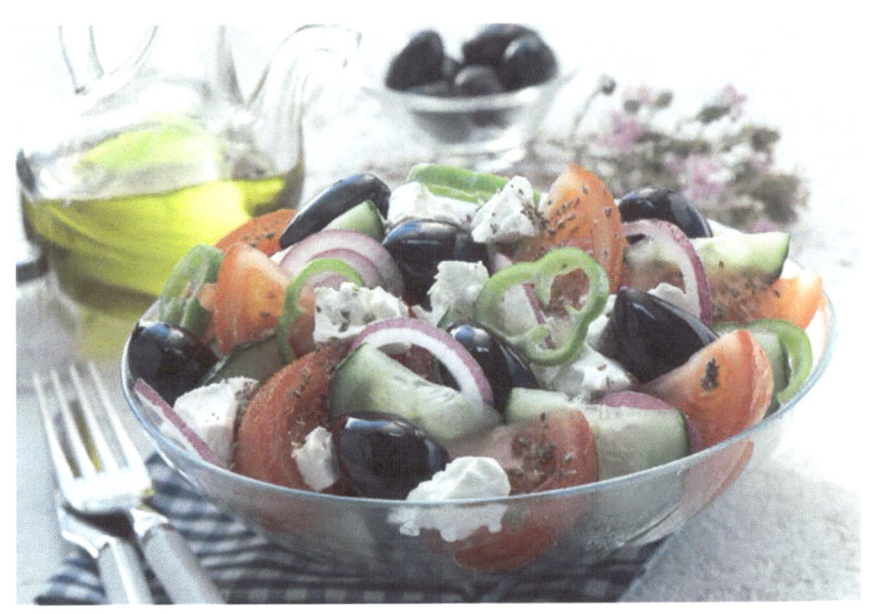

You have created one of the most easy, delicious and healthy dishes/salads in the world.

All that's left is to try your masterpiece and you will remember why I said it is important to add it to your nutrition/diet!

Moreover, if you do add it, you will notice significant boost in your energy, an valuable increase in body and mind performance.

One other secret is to eat the salad right after you prepare it. It takes 5-10 minutes to prepare the salad if you have all the ingredients gathered...

Here, I must close this guide which I hope you enjoyed and found useful...

It would be even more fulfilling for me, if you try this authentic Greek salad recipe and see it's effects for yourself.

Here is some more advice...:

1. Always eat this salad along with a slice (or 2!) of fresh or toasted bread and make sure there's no olive oil left in the salad plate when you are done eating... ☺

2. Always eat a Greek Salad before you drink alcohol. The oil will protect your stomach and along with the Feta Cheese will help alcohol be absorbed smoothly and it will give you a sweet whirl (tizzy). And of course consume 10 times more water than alcohol while drinking...

3. **If you want to strengthen your bones and your memory** then try to find a source for original Greek Feta Cheese and use a minimum of 2 descent pieces (1 for each person)

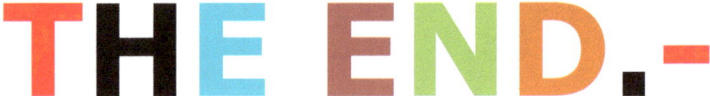

THE END.-

Promotional Resources

Herbs, oils and other aphrodisiacs! Highly recommended, please visit:
http://hyperdeals.biz/go/17/

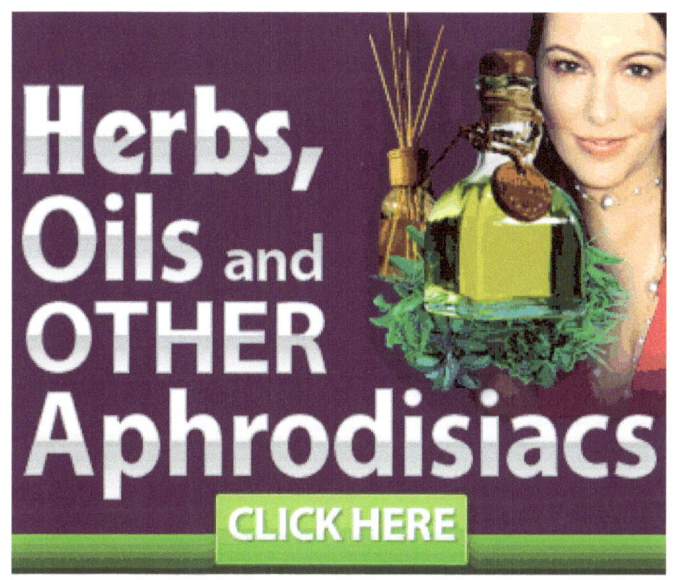

More aphrodisiac offers? See this:
http://aphrodisiac.webs.com/apps/links/

Learn all the secrets of Wines. Become a wine expert, click to explore more:
http://hyperdeals.biz/go/14/

Credits

To my lovely co-author Maria Markella who helped my beyond any extend.
Look at her books:

http://amazon.com/author/mariamarkella

All images from Wikimedia Commons:
http://commons.wikimedia.org

Promotional materials, logos and images belong to their respective owner.

For any issues concerning copyright or this little cook-book please contact me:
lazageo@gmail.com

MORE NOTES:

>>>> Would you like to see more of my books? Visit this link:

http://amazon.com/author/lazarosgeorgoulas

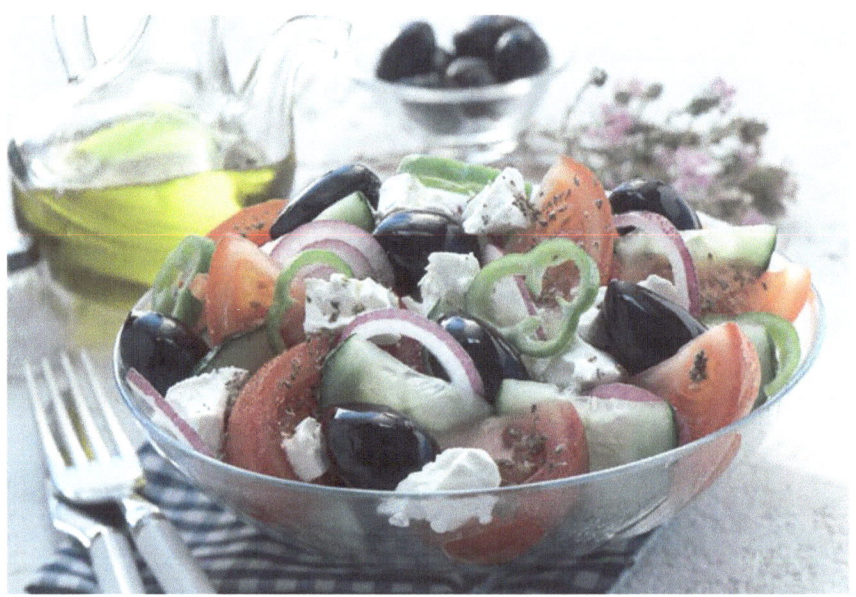

www.ingramcontent.com/pod-product-compliance
Lightning Source LLC
Chambersburg PA
CBHW051128290526
45796CB00001B/7